Women and Nutrition

i

Women and Nutrition
Candy Cumming, MS, RD

Publisher: Robert H. Garrison, Jr., MA, RPh
Editor In Chief: Elizabeth Somer, MA, RD
Managing Editor: Lisa M. Moye
Editorial Director: Janet L. Haley
Art Director: Scott Mayeda
Production Directors: Jeff Elkind, Irene Villa
Copy Editors: Norma Trost Foor, Jean Forsythe, Mary Houser,
          Stephen C. Schneider, R. H. Garrison, Sr., RPh
Cover Design: Stefanko & Hetz, Jeff Elkind
Photography: Bob and Irene Nishihira, Carlsbad, CA
Illustration: Scott Mayeda, Walter Stuart, Jennifer Hewitson

Health Media of America, Inc., has made every effort to ensure the accuracy of the information herein. For individual application, treatment suggestions must be considered in light of the individual's health, subject to a physician's specific recommendations. The authors, editors, and the publisher cannot be held responsible for any undetected errors found in this book.

**Revised Edition Published 1988 by
Grolier Educational Corporation, Danbury, CT, 06816**

Printed in the United States of America.

ISBN 0-7172-7129-3

Contents

Introduction

Introduction

The majority of women today are employed outside of the home. More than 60% of American women 20 to 64 years old have or are actively seeking paying jobs.[1] As a result of this shift away from homemaking, more meals are eaten away from home and carry-out foods, fast foods, and convenience foods are becoming increasingly popular. While food preparation might not be as time-consuming as it has been for generations, women must not overlook their unique nutritional needs.

Pregnant women have special nutritional requirements. The demands of a growing fetus increase the need for many vital nutrients. The same is true during breastfeeding.

Many other situations such as menstruation, weight control, use of contraceptives, and the hormonal changes of menopause also have an impact on nutritional status.

The risk of many diseases, such as osteoporosis and cancers of the female reproductive system, is increased when diets are composed of fatty foods and lack sufficient amounts of foods rich in vitamins and minerals. In addition, the added stress of balancing a career and family life also might influence nutritional needs.

National nutrition surveys show that women might not be consuming adequate amounts of some nutrients. Marginal intakes of vitamin A, vitamin C, vitamin B_6, calcium, iron, and magnesium are common in many women's diets. The diets of women also might be low in chromium and folic acid. Limited food intake and an average consumption of less than 1,800 calories is a primary contributor to nutrient deficiencies. Many of these nutrient deficiencies are related to diseases common in women such as anemia, breast cancer, osteoporosis, and Premenstrual Syndrome.[2-5]

Diet is one of the most important contributors to the health and well-being of women according to The Surgeon General's Report "Healthy People" and the National Academy of Sciences.[6,7] How a woman handles her family and/or a career will depend, at least in part, on her nutritional vitality. If she is adequately nourished, she has a greater chance of obtaining the most enjoyment out of work and home life.

WOMEN AND NUTRITION provides information on specific health and nutritional issues related to women's needs. Practical, simple guidelines for healthy eating are given and suggestions are provided for quick and easy ways to meet nutritional needs throughout a lifetime.

1
Anemia:
Do Women
Have Tired Blood?

Some women suffer from chronic fatigue. They tire easily, feel weak, or have difficulty concentrating and have an insufficient amount of energy to carry out their responsibilities. Many conditions can cause fatigue, however, a common cause in women is anemia, sometimes referred to as "tired blood."

Anemia is a reduction in the number, color, or size of red blood cells. Red blood cells carry oxygen from the lungs to the tissues and transport carbon dioxide, a waste product, from the tissues to the lungs to be exhaled. Any condition that reduces the oxygen-carrying capacity of red blood cells would reduce the oxygen supply to tissues, including the brain and muscles. Symptoms would include lethargy, poor concentration, and weakness.

Anemia can result from physical conditions, such as acute blood loss from excessive bleeding or chronic low-grade blood loss from a bleeding ulcer. Poor dietary intake or absorption of iron, vitamin B_{12}, vitamin B_6, vitamin C, or copper can also result in anemia. The most common nutritional anemias are caused by a deficiency of iron or folic acid. Iron is a mineral in hemoglobin, a protein found in red blood cells. An insufficient iron supply means less

1

oxygen is delivered to the tissues. As a result, a person tires quickly, feels lethargic, or does not concentrate well. Other nutrients involved in the production of hemoglobin or maintenance of red blood cells include protein, copper, vitamin E, vitamin B_6, folic acid, vitamin B_{12}, and other B vitamins. *(Figure 1)*

Most women do not consume adequate amounts of iron.[9] The main reason for a poor dietary intake of iron is limited food consumption. There are only 6 grams of iron in every 1,000 calories of well-selected foods and a menstruating woman must eat 3,000 calories to meet her daily iron requirement of 18 mg.[9,10] Many women consume only 1,500 to 1,600 calories a day.[5] Many eat less calories in an effort

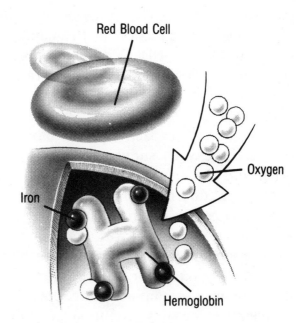

Red Blood Cell

Oxygen

Iron

Hemoglobin

Figure 1. The Red Blood Cell

to lose weight. Adequate iron intake is difficult, if not impossible, on such a limited food intake.[8,9]

Several factors influence a low calorie intake, including a sedentary lifestyle that does not demand a lot of calories to maintain weight, restrictive weight control diets, and fewer calories needed than men to maintain a smaller body size and muscle mass.

In addition to an inadequate iron intake, women have an increased requirement for iron. Menstrual losses averaged throughout the month constitute a daily iron loss of about 1.0 mg or a 28 mg loss of iron each month. The demands of pregnancy include an increased need for iron of about 500 mg to 1,000 mg. Lactation (breastfeeding) depletes the body of 1.0 mg to 2.5 mg of iron each day.[11]

Postmenopausal women have lower iron requirements because they do not have menstrual blood losses. Their need for iron is 10 mg a day and can be supplied by a well-chosen diet that supplies at least 1,500 calories.[10]

Iron Deficiency And Anemia: Are They The Same?

Not all women have "tired blood," or iron deficiency anemia. A woman does not have to be anemic to be deficient in iron. Anemia is one of the later stages of iron deficiency and denotes long-term iron deficiency. Prior to anemia, the body's stores of iron have first been depleted, followed by a reduction in blood cell formation. During these stages the symptoms are vague and develop gradually and the deficiency can go undetected.

As many as two-thirds of all menstruating women and a majority of pregnant women have little or no stores of iron in their tissues and are in the first stages of iron depletion.[10,12] At this point hemoglobin levels are still adequate. A woman with low iron stores and normal hemoglobin levels is likely to become anemic with the added demands of pregnancy. Blood loss, whether a result of donation, hemorrhage, internal bleeding, or use of an intrauterine device (increases menstrual blood loss), places further strain on the body's need for iron. Heavy athletic training can result in additional iron losses in perspiration.[13]

Symptoms Of Iron Deficiency

General fatigue is the most common symptom of iron deficiency. In addition, a woman might appear pale, have headaches, have poor concentration and increased susceptibility to infection and disease, feel lethargic or weak, have a poor appetite, or be short of breath. Gastrointestinal complaints are also possible.[8,11]

Signs of long-standing iron deficiency include a craving for ice or other non-food items.[11] A smooth tongue and cracking at the corners of the mouth might signal iron deficiency, or might indicate other problems.

Iron deficiency also leads to lusterless, brittle, ridged fingernails. Eventually, nails become concave, a situation known as "spooning."[10,14]

Untreated anemia can result in respiratory changes and heart failure.[8]

Regular medical checkups that include a blood test for iron status are important since a deficiency can go undetected until the later stages. The blood test should include a hematocrit, which is a test for the amount of red blood cells per unit of blood, and hemoglobin, which is a test for the amount of hemoglobin in a given amount of blood. These measurements are only accurate in diagnosing the final stages of iron deficiency. Measurements of serum (a portion of blood) transferrin saturation, serum ferritin concentration, and/or iron-binding capacity can be done; these blood tests are more sensitive than hemoglobin levels in detecting earlier stages of iron deficiency.[12] *(Figure 2, Page 6)*

Improving Iron Intake

The prevention and treatment of iron deficiency begins with an increase in iron intake from diet and supplement sources. The estimated iron needs of most women is about 1.8 mg a day and since only about 10% of the dietary iron is absorbed this accounts for the Recommended Dietary Allowance (RDA) of 18 mg.

A simple way to increase iron in the diet is to use iron cookware, especially when cooking foods that are acidic. For example, the iron content of spaghetti sauce can increase from 3 mg to 87 mg per 3 1/2 ounce serving by using an iron pot.[15]

Factors Influencing Iron Absorption

How much iron a woman absorbs from a meal is not equal to the amount present in the food. It depends upon the kind of iron in the food as well as other food substances that influence iron absorption.[16]

Iron is found in two forms: heme iron (the iron found in meats) and non-heme iron (the iron found in cereals, dried beans and peas, fruits, and vegetables). Heme iron contributes a minor amount of iron

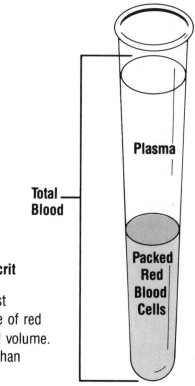

Figure 2. The Hematocrit

The hematocrit blood test measures the percentage of red blood cells to total blood volume. In women, a value less than 37% indicates anemia.

to the total diet. Even diets that contain a large portion of meat derive only 10% to 15% of the total iron intake from heme iron. However, heme iron is well absorbed and between 10% and 35% of the total ingested crosses the intestinal barrier and enters the blood stream. Non-heme iron or iron from plant sources constitutes a large portion of the daily iron intake but is poorly absorbed; only about 2% to 10% is absorbed from the diet. Because non-heme iron is a major portion of the daily iron intake, anything that will increase its absorption is important.[11]

Heme iron in foods from animal sources increases the absorption of non-heme iron when the two are eaten together. The percentage of iron absorbed from kidney beans increases as much as four-fold when the beans are consumed with a small amount of chicken or lean beef.[17] Chinese food that combines small amounts of meat with large amounts of vegetables, or Italian food that combines a small amount of meat with a generous portion of pasta are examples of foods that combine heme iron and non-heme iron to increase iron absorption. *(Figure 3)*

Some dietary factors hinder iron absorption while others assist it. Foods high in vitamin C increase the absorption of both heme and non-heme iron. However, the inclusion of black tea or the additive ethylenediamine tetraacetic acid (EDTA) with a meal can reduce the availability of non-heme iron by 50%.[8] EDTA is added to a variety of foods including salad dressings, margarine, canned shellfish, and some processed fruits and vegetables. Eggs, soy products, and coffee also inhibit iron absorption. Another dietary factor that limits iron availability is phytate, a substance found in whole wheat. When whole wheat is leavened, as in yeast bread, the interfering effect

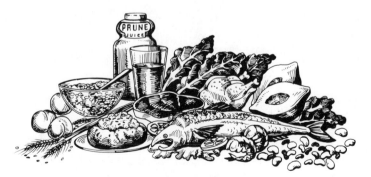

Figure 3. Foods High In Iron

of the phytate is reduced. This makes regular whole wheat bread superior to unleavened varieties.[16]

To increase iron absorption from foods:

- include a vitamin C food with every meal;
- include a small amount of lean meat, chicken, or fish with meals;
- avoid drinking tea or coffee with meals;
- avoid foods that contain EDTA;
- increase consumption of iron-rich foods; and
- cook in iron pots.

The iron in supplements and fortified foods is not well absorbed. A serving of fortified cereal can contain 10 mg to 18 mg of iron, however, the form of iron is so poorly absorbed that very little is used by the body.[16]

Large doses of iron taken on an empty stomach might cause stomach upsets such as nausea, distention, constipation or diarrhea, and heartburn. These symptoms might be relieved by beginning supplementation with a small dose of iron and increasing the dose slowly over several days or weeks.[8]

When iron status has been low it will take between one to three weeks of supplementation and increased dietary intake of iron for improvement. The first sign of improvement is an increase in red blood cells. An individual should continue to monitor the iron content of the diet for 6 to 12 months after normal blood levels of iron and red blood cells have been restored. This continued intake will allow iron stores to be replenished.

A physician should be consulted if anemia is suspected and iron supplementation is initiated. Iron poisoning is possible when excessive amounts of iron are consumed.[8,18] As a preventive measure, however, supplementing daily with 18 mg, the Recommended Dietary Allowance (RDA), might be beneficial.

Folic Acid, Vitamin B$_{12}$, And Anemia

A deficiency of folic acid or vitamin B$_{12}$ can result from a diet that is low in dark green leafy vegetables or foods from animal sources, poor absorption, or increased nutrient requirements. Body stores of folic acid are depleted within weeks when the diet is low in this B vitamin.[8] In addition, national surveys show the folic acid content of the American diet is about half of the suggested amount.[4] A vitamin B$_{12}$ deficiency is less likely to occur since the body can store months or years worth of this vitamin.

Folic acid and vitamin B$_{12}$ are necessary for normal cell development. An inadequate daily intake of either vitamin results in impaired red blood cell formation. The red blood cells do not develop properly. They are fragile, easily broken, and are inefficient at carrying oxygen to the tissues. The result is anemia.

Adequate dietary intake of these B vitamins is essential to prevent deficiencies. Folic acid is of particular concern since the vitamin is found primarily in spinach, chard, collard greens, broccoli, and other dark green leafy vegetables and in orange juice. These foods are often ignored in the daily diet. *(Table 1, Page 10)*

Folic acid is easily destroyed by prolonged storage, light, heat in cooking or processing, and is lost when cooking water is discarded. Reheating of vegetables causes further destruction of folic acid. Fruits and vegetables should be eaten fresh, with minimal cooking or storage.

Table 1	Folic Acid Content Of Selected Foods	
Food **(Serving Size)**		**Folic Acid** **(mcg)**
Spinach, cooked (1 cup)		164
Orange juice, frozen (1 cup)		136
Beets, cooked (1 cup)		133
Wheat germ, toasted (1/4 cup)		118
Pinto beans, cooked (1 cup)		112
Broccoli, cooked (1 spear)		101
Romaine lettuce, raw (1 cup)		98
Peas, frozen (1 cup)		77
Tomatoes, raw (1 med.)		53
Cantaloupe (1/4 med.)		42

Vitamin B_{12} intake should be adequate if low-fat dairy foods or other foods from animal sources are consumed frequently. Vegetarians who do not consume foods from animal sources and people who lack Intrinsic Factor, a substance in the stomach that increases vitamin B_{12} absorption, are at risk for vitamin B_{12} deficiency.[8] Seniors are especially susceptible to vitamin B_{12} deficiency. A daily source of the vitamin can be obtained from soymilk fortified with vitamin B_{12} or from supplements.

2
Premenstrual Syndrome

Premenstrual syndrome (PMS) includes the anxiety, depression, food cravings, and bloated feeling experienced before the beginning of menstruation.

The term "premenstrual syndrome" is used to describe a wide variety of physical and emotional symptoms experienced by women. More than 150 symptoms are attributed to this disorder. Usually these symptoms occur 1 to 14 days before the menstrual period begins and are followed by a symptom-free phase once the period is over.[19]

For years women's complaints about premenstrual changes, however mild or severe, were ignored. Women were told these difficulties were all in their heads, a frustrating response to an already-frustrating problem. Current research shows that there is a physiological basis to PMS. Although a single cause of PMS has not been found, scientists suggest that PMS is caused by a complex interplay of hormonal imbalances, stress, and nutritional deficiencies.

The female hormones, estrogen and progesterone, might be involved in this disorder. PMS might be caused by a deficiency of the hormone progesterone.[20] Other researchers have noted an imbalance in the relationship between estrogen and progesterone.

It is thought that excess estrogen remains in the bloodstream as a result of the liver's inability to

11

break down estrogen because of a shortage of B vitamins.[19] A recent study found that nutritional supplementation was able to balance the ratio between these two hormones, and PMS symptoms were reduced or eliminated.[21,22] Excess estrogen also can remain in the bloodstream when there is a decreased amount of estrogen excreted.[23] A high fiber diet, because it assists estrogen excretion, is recommended for women troubled by PMS.[24] *(Figure 4)*

Who Has PMS?

Any menstruating woman is a candidate for PMS, with nearly 50% of all women in their childbearing years experiencing moderate or severe symptoms. Even though adolescents may suffer from it, symptoms of PMS are more severe as a woman gets older. Often women in their 30s notice premenstrual difficulties for the first time.[25]

PMS might begin after a significant hormonal event, such as puberty or after use of the birth control pill, a period of amenorrhea (failure to menstruate),

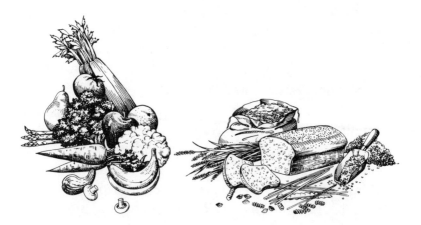

Figure 4. Fiber Foods

12

or pregnancy. Women with a history of toxemia during pregnancy have a 90% chance of developing PMS compared to a 30% chance for women without toxemia. Sterilization, especially tubal ligation, often triggers premenstrual symptoms.[19]

A variety of lifestyle factors seem to make symptoms worse including stress, an inadequate amount of outdoor physical activity, and a diet that is high in sugar and refined carbohydrates, salt, fat, alcohol, and caffeine.[19]

Although most women experience symptoms before menstruation, many are not aware that they have premenstrual syndrome. Often women accept the effects of PMS as part of being a woman and cope with their symptoms. Keeping a calendar of body and mood changes is the best way to determine if the symptoms a woman experiences occur during the two weeks prior to the period and are associated with PMS. *(Table 2, Page 14)*

Premenstrual Symptoms

Four major symptom groups of PMS have been identified. A woman might experience symptoms in one or several groups.

1. Premenstrual Tension is characterized by nervous tension, mood swings, irritability and anxiety.
2. Hyperhydration, or the hyperhydration syndrome, is marked by weight gain, swelling in the hands and feet, breast tenderness, and abdominal bloating.
3. Cravings mean an increase in appetite with cravings for sweets or salty foods. Symptoms also include headache, fatigue, dizziness, and a pounding heart.

13

Table 2 Menstrual Symptom Diary (MSD)

NAME: _____ AGE: _____ HEIGHT: _____ WEIGHT: _____

Grading of Menses: 0-none; **1**-slight; **2**-moderate; he**heavy**; **4**-heavy and clots.

Day #1 is the first day of menstruation

Grading of Symptoms, (complaints) 0-none; **1**-mild-present but does not interfere with activities; **2**-moderate-present and interferes with activities but not disabling. **3**-Unable to function.

	1	2	3	4	5	6	7	8	9	10	11	12	13	14	15	16	17	18	19	20	21	22	23	24	25	26	27	28	29	30
Day of cycle																														
Date																														
Menses																														
Premenstrual Tension Nervous tension																														
Mood swings																														
Irritability																														
Anxiety																														
Hyperhydration Weight gain																														
Swelling of extremeties																														
Breast tenderness																														
Abdominal bloating																														
Cravings Headache																														
Craving for sweets																														
Increased appetite																														
Heart pounding																														
Fatigue																														
Dizziness or faintness																														
Depression Depression																														
Forgetfulness																														
Crying																														
Confusion																														
Insomnia																														

14

4. Depression is also common and includes forgetfulness, crying, confusion, and insomnia.[25]

Over 150 symptoms have been associated with PMS, however, and the sequence and combination of symptoms can vary between women. For instance, some women have acne flare-ups right before their periods. Others are constipated. Some women experience nausea when they exercise. The type and severity of symptoms also might vary each month and might reflect lifestyle changes or stress.

Stress: Stress and nutrition are related. Stress increases the excretion of magnesium and raises the requirement for this nutrient.[26] The theory that a magnesium deficiency contributes to PMS is supported by the finding that women with PMS often have low blood levels of magnesium.[27]

Sugar: In studies of the dietary patterns of women with PMS compared to the diets of women who are not disturbed by this problem, women with PMS consume more sugar, averaging approximately 20 teaspoons a day. Excessive sugar consumption contributes to a magnesium deficiency because the body needs magnesium to metabolize sugar. At the same time, sugar does not provide magnesium.[28] *(Table 3, Page 16)*

Vitamins: Women who supplement their diets with the B complex vitamins usually are less likely to be disturbed by PMS.[28]

A Nutritional Program For PMS

Vitamin B$_6$: Supplementation with vitamin B$_6$ might relieve premenstrual symptoms in some women. One study found that supplements of vitamin B$_6$, taken daily from the tenth day of one cycle until the third

Table 3   Sugar In The Diet

Food	Portion	Tablespoons*/ Portion
Cake, iced	1 piece	🥄🥄🥄🥄
Ice cream sundae	1	🥄🥄🥄🥄
Jello	1 cup	🥄🥄🥄
Pie, fruit	1 slice	🥄🥄🥄
Soda	12 oz.	🥄🥄🥄
Donut, glazed	1	🥄🥄
Fruit "drink"	8 oz.	🥄🥄
Lemonade	8 oz.	🥄🥄
Pie, custard	1 slice	🥄🥄
Popsicle	1 twin bar	🥄🥄
Sherbet	1/2 cup	🥄🥄
Yogurt, flavored	8 oz.	🥄🥄
Candy bar	1 average	🥄
Cereal, presweetened	1/2 cup	🥄
Cookies	2 small	🥄
Donut, plain	1	🥄
Fruit, canned	1/2 cup	🥄
Ice cream	1/2 cup	🥄
Jelly, marmalade, jam	1 Tbsp	🥄
Milk, chocolate	8 oz.	🥄
Pudding	1/2 cup	🥄
Roll, sweet	1	🥄
Sugar	1 Tbsp	🥄
Syrup	1 Tbsp	🥄

*1 Tbsp = 3 teaspoons

16

day of the next, was effective in the treatment of PMS.[29] This supports earlier work that suggested vitamin B_6 is effective in the treatment of PMS and should be considered as a therapeutic agent.[30]

Vitamin B_6 works with magnesium by helping transport the mineral into cells. Supplemental B_6 might raise the level of magnesium inside red blood cells.[31]

Self-medication with vitamin B_6 can be harmful because at large doses the vitamin is toxic. Women who take more than 500 mg of vitamin B_6 daily for a prolonged period might have nerve damage with symptoms that include difficulty walking and a numbness and tingling in their hands and feet. Vitamin B_6 at doses above 100 mg a day should be taken with the supervision of a physician.[29,32,33]

Fats and Evening Primrose Oil: High levels of essential fatty acids, such as linoleic acid, are sometimes found in the blood of women with PMS. This condition might be caused by an inability to convert this essential fat into the prostaglandin, PGE_1, which has a favorable effect on PMS symptoms.[34]

A prostaglandin is a hormone-like substance that regulates numerous biological functions and is formed from dietary fats. The prostaglandin PGE_1 reduces water retention and other symptoms such as headaches, heart pounding, fainting, increased appetite, and food cravings. PGE_1 is formed in the body from vegetable oils. However, the conversion from oil to prostaglandin requires magnesium, zinc, vitamin C, and several B-complex vitamins. If any nutrient is deficient, prostaglandin synthesis will not proceed normally.[25]

The use of evening primrose oil has been suggested for PMS since this oil contains gamma linolenic acid (GLA), a fatty acid that is produced as an intermediate step in the production of prostaglandins. Supplements of GLA might benefit those people with faulty prostaglandin production.[35]

Considering the relationship between magnesium and vitamin B_6, as well as vitamin B_6's dependency on other vitamins in the B-complex, and the relationship of certain vitamins and minerals to prostaglandin production, a nutritional supplementation program for PMS might include a well-balanced multivitamin-mineral supplement.[22]

Women troubled by PMS might improve their symptoms by making the following dietary changes:[24,25]

- Reducing sugar intake,
- Increasing fiber,
- Including 1 to 2 tablespoons of safflower oil in the diet,
- Reducing fat intake,
- Reducing salt intake if fluid retention is a problem,
- And avoiding caffeine, especially when anxiety and breast tenderness are problems.

In addition:

- Include physical activity in the daily routine, and
- Practice stress reduction techniques regularly.

Many women have found relief with this moderate lifestyle approach and it is recommended for the initial treatment of premenstrual syndrome. A physician should be consulted if symptoms persist, since hormone and/or drug therapy might be indicated.[36]

3
Oral Contraceptives And Nutrition

Although oral contraceptives provide an easy-to-use, effective form of birth control, they do have health and nutritional side effects.[11,37]

Hypertension (high blood pressure) is a possible side effect of this form of birth control. Oral contraceptive-induced hypertension occurs in women who have a family history of hypertension, as well as in women who have had problems with blood pressure before using the Pill.

Individuals who are predisposed to diabetes are more likely to develop diabetes when using birth control pills. The most serious side effect is the possibility of blood clots in the lungs, brain, or cardiovascular system. This can happen in relatively young women, especially in heavy smokers.[38] *(Table 4, Page 20)*

Vitamins, Minerals, And Oral Contraceptives

Vitamin B$_6$: Researchers have investigated the effects of oral contraceptives on nutritional status. The daily requirement for vitamin B$_6$ is increased by the hormone estrogen used in oral contraceptives.

A deficiency of vitamin B$_6$ caused by oral contraceptives might cause depression. An increased intake of vitamin B$_6$ from food or supplements might improve the depression experienced by some women

19

Table 4	Side Effects Of Oral Contraceptives
	Blood clots in the legs, pelvis, lungs, heart, or brain
	Headaches
	Blurred vision, loss of vision, or flashing lights
	Chest pains or shortness of breath
	Nausea
	Weight gain, fluid retention, breast fullness or tenderness
	Mild headaches
	Spotting between periods
	Decreased menstrual blood flow
	Missed periods
	Yeast infection, vaginal itching, or discharge
	Depression, mood changes, fatigue

using the Pill.[39] A daily intake of 1.5 mg to 5 mg of vitamin B_6 is usually suggested for women on oral contraceptives.[40]

Vitamin B_1 and Vitamin B_2: Oral contraceptives might have a negative effect on vitamin B_1 and vitamin B_2, especially in women who already are low in these two B vitamins. Inclusion of several servings a day of foods rich in these vitamins would help counteract the medication-induced deficiency.

Vitamin B_1 is found in whole wheat and enriched breads and cereals, lean pork, lean beef, nuts, and dried beans and peas. The best dietary sources of vitamin B_2 are low-fat dairy foods, such as low-fat and nonfat milk, low-fat cheeses, and low-fat yogurt. Other dietary sources include broccoli, mushrooms, and dark green leafy vegetables.

Folic Acid: A localized deficiency of folic acid is sometimes found in cervical tissue. This deficiency might be the result of dietary intake, hormonal stimulation of cervical tissue, or other stresses. In one study, about 20% of women using oral contraceptives had enlarged cervical and vaginal cells. After receiving folic acid supplementation, the condition was corrected in all cases.[41,42] Cervical dysplasia, (a condition that can be precancerous), might be associated with a localized folic acid deficiency and this deficiency might be corrected by an increased intake of folic acid.[43]

Not all women on oral contraceptives need to take a folic acid supplement. All diets, however, should contain at least one serving a day of folic acid-rich foods such as dark green vegetables. Additional food sources of folic acid include dried beans and peas, nuts, fresh oranges, and whole wheat products.

Zinc: Absorption of folic acid is dependent on zinc. If zinc is inadequately supplied, an intestinal enzyme involved in the absorption of folic acid will not function properly and this might lead to a folic acid deficiency.[44] Zinc is found in dried beans and peas, lean meats, nuts and seeds, poultry, shellfish, milk, cheese, and whole grain breads and cereals.

Vitamin A: Oral contraceptives might increase blood levels of vitamin A by causing the release of the vitamin from liver storage, which depletes vitamin A in the liver. Women who take oral contraceptives should consume adequate amounts of vitamin A from dark green and orange vegetables and fruits, vitamin A-fortified milk, or supplements.[45]

Iron: On the positive side, oral contraceptive use reduces blood loss during menstruation. This suggests that the iron needs of women on the Pill might be reduced and a woman would be at reduced risk for iron deficiency anemia.[45]

4
Cancer And Related Disorders

Fibrocystic Breast Disease

Some women experience lumps and pain in the breasts. Although this condition may be constant, it is often cyclical and worsens prior to the onset of menstruation. For years this condition was called fibrocystic breast disease. However, the usefulness of this diagnosis is questionable since the term is often used as a catch-all for a variety of breast conditions. Fibrocystic breast disease, mammary dysplasia, cystic mastalgia, and benign breast disease are a few of the terms used to describe this disorder.[46,47]

In clinical terms, fibrocysts are fluid-filled sacs surrounded by fibrous tissue. Many women with discomfort and symptoms are not told the type of cyst or mass they have, because it is not cancer. *(Figure 5, Page 24)*

Fibrocystic breast disease has been linked to an increased risk for developing breast cancer, a disease that occures in one out of every eleven women in the United States.[48] However, researchers now believe that 70% of the women with fibrocystic breast disease should not be concerned about an increased cancer risk. The remaining 30% of these women have double the risk. A small percentage of women (4%) have atypical breast lesions with an abnormal structure that looks like cancer. Women who have atypical lesions or who have a family history of breast cancer have 11 times the risk of developing

23

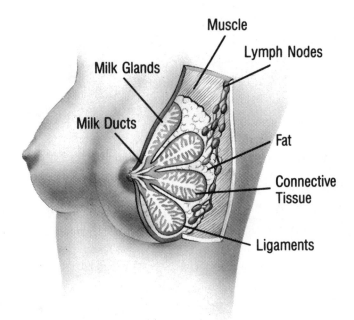

Figure 5. Normal Breast Tissue

Breast tissue is a complex structure that undergoes continual changes throughout the menstrual cycle in preparation for possible pregnancy.

breast cancer as women with neither of these risk factors.[46,47]

Fibrocystic breast disease includes a variety of disorders, only a few of which increase a woman's risk for developing cancer. Any mass in the breast that is not cancerous is called a benign breast lump.

Whether or not fibrocystic breasts are classified as "diseased" is only one concern for women who deal with the associated lumps and pain. The problem with the bumpiness is that it makes it more difficult to detect a cancerous lump. The problem with the associated discomfort is that the breasts can be tender and any type of pressure is painful.

Until recently, treatment for mild fibrocystic breasts did not exist. Surgery was reserved for severe cases. Prevention and treatment suggestions now are available to help reduce the incidence and severity of this disorder. Dietary suggestions include a decrease in methylxanthines and dietary fat and an increase in vitamin E.

Methylxanthines: The elimination of methylxanthines from the diet might treat fibrocystic breast disease. Methylxanthines include caffeine in coffee, tea, some soft drinks, and some drugs; theobromine in chocolate, tea, and some soft drinks; and theophylline in tea. *(Table 5)*

Coffee consumption is often moderate to high in the diets of women with fibrocystic breast disease. When coffee and other foods or drugs that contain

Table 5	Methylxanthines In Food		
Product	Caffeine (mgs)	Theobromine (mgs)	Theophylline (mgs)
Coffee (5 oz.)			
Dripolator	150	3.5	1
Instant	66	1.5	tr
Decaf Brewed	4.5	tr	tr
Soft Drinks (12 oz.)	34–61	tr	tr
Brewed Tea	45	9	6
Cocoa (5 oz.)	13	173	tr
Drugs	16–200	—	—

tr = less than 1 milligram per serving

methylxanthines are eliminated from the diet breast lumps and pain often are reduced or eliminated within 6 months.

Other lifestyle factors influence the effectiveness of a methylxanthine-free diet in reducing fibrocystic breast disease. For example, women who smoke do not show any progress until they quit smoking and follow a methylxanthine-restricted diet.[47]

Preliminary evidence shows that the elimination of all products containing methylxanthines for six to eight weeks might be an effective treatment for fibrocystic breast disease. If the lumps and pain do not disappear, a physician should be consulted and a biopsy should be done to determine if the lumps are malignant (cancerous) or benign (non-cancerous).[49]

It is thought that benign breast lumps are the result of an accumulation of body chemicals. Under normal conditions, these chemicals do not accumulate because an enzyme deactivates them. Methylxanthines inhibit the action of this enzyme. In an analysis of the composition of benign breast lumps, levels of these chemicals are 50% higher than in normal breast tissue; malignant breast tissues have higher levels.[49]

The caffeine/methylxanthine-fibrocystic breast disease link is controversial. However, research continues to substantiate the preliminary findings and women continue to report a reduction in symptoms.[50,51]

Any woman with breast lumps and pain can eliminate these foods. Giving up caffeine and its associated substances is not harmful to health and might be beneficial.[52,53]

Vitamin E: An adequate intake of vitamin E might relieve symptoms and normalize abnormal hormonal patterns observed in some women with fibrocystic breast disease.[54]

Vitamin E is found in vegetable oils and is abundant in safflower oil. Substantial amounts of vitamin E are lost in the heat processing and bleaching of commercial vegetable oils.[55] Cold pressed vegetable oils might contain more of the vitamin. Other dietary sources of vitamin E include nuts, seeds, wheat germ oil, whole grain breads and cereals, and dark green leafy vegetables.

Dietary Fat: A reduction in dietary fat intake might prevent or treat this condition. When dietary fat is reduced to 20% of the total calories, in contrast to the typical 42%, breast pain decreases and blood levels of the female hormones estrogen and prolactin decline. A decline in these hormones is associated with a reduced risk for cancer.[56,57]

Breast Cancer

Breast cancer is the leading cause of death among women who are 40 to 49 years old. There are ways a woman can reduce the risk for developing breast cancer.[58]

Dietary Fat: The death rate from breast cancer increases as the consumption of dietary fat increases.[58,59]

High-fat diets encourage the development of breast tumors. Excessive fat consumption alters the relationship between female hormones, which might transform a benign breast cyst or lump into a cancerous one.[57,58]

While it is inappropriate to say that excess fat causes cancer, evidence suggests that fat can alter hormonal metabolism and create an environment that is more susceptible to cancer. Additionally, high-fat diets adversely affect the immune system.[60-62]

High-fat diets hasten the development of breast cancer when compared to low-fat diets.

Fat intake should be maintained below 30% of the day's total calories.[63,64] Ounce for ounce, fat supplies more than twice the amount of calories as carbohydrates (sugar and starch) or protein. It is easy for the percentage of fat calories to exceed the 30% guideline unless careful attention is paid to hidden fats. For example, whole milk supplies 50% of its total calories from fat. Lowfat, or 2% lowfat milk, is 34% fat calories. Nonfat milk is less than 0.5% fat calories and contains the same amount of protein, minerals, and vitamins. Hamburger is considered a protein food, but over 60% of its calories can come from fat. A baked potato has trace amounts of fat; sour cream and butter can increase the fat calories a hundred-fold. To reduce the fat in the diet:

- Use nonfat or low-fat milk.
- Reduce fat in recipes to one-third.
- Bake, steam, broil, or poach foods.
- Skim fat from homemade soup stock.
- Baste foods with lemon, tomato juice, fruit juice, nonfat milk, low-salt soy sauce, cooking wines, or spices.
- Use imitation mayonnaise and mix with equal portions of nonfat yogurt.
- Saute foods in defatted chicken stock and use non-stick pans.
- Use low-calorie jam on toast, instead of butter.
- Use nonfat milk for creamed soups, sauces, or gravies.
- Use nonfat yogurt with a dash of lemon for dips.
- Use 99% fat free or low-fat cottage cheese.
- Use tuna packed in water.

- Select chives, nonfat yogurt, or cottage cheese as toppings for baked potatoes.
- Choose sherbet, ice milk, or sorbet instead of ice cream.
- Choose bagels or whole wheat rolls instead of doughnuts and breakfast rolls.
- Snack on unbuttered popcorn, rye crisp crackers, fresh fruits, and vegetables, rather than chips and nuts.

Obesity: Excessive body fat, particularly in post-menopausal women, increases the risk of developing cancer.[58] The death rates from breast cancer, and cancers of the endometrium (lining of the uterus), cervix, and uterus are higher in women who are 40% or more overweight. After menopause excess body fat increases the risk of developing breast cancer. A postmenopausal, obese woman has nearly 12 times the risk of a lean, premenopausal woman for the development of breast cancer.[65]

Compared to other women with breast cancer, obese women develop breast cancer earlier in life. In addition, heavy women who undergo a mastectomy do not survive as long as women who are at or near their ideal body weight. Weight loss is recommended for all women, but especially those who have already had breast cancer.[57,65]

It appears that obesity increases the body's production of estrogen by fat cells, the liver, and the brain. The excessive production of estrogen creates a hormonal imbalance that is associated with an increased risk for cancer. Clearing this excessive estrogen out of the body might reduce cancer risk. Dietary fiber, which assists the excretion of estrogen, might provide some protection. Women who consume a high-fiber vegetarian diet excrete more estrogen and might be at lower risk for breast cancer. Women who are vegetarians consume an average of 28 grams of fiber a day compared to only 12 grams by women eating the traditional American diet.[23,65] *(Figure 6)*

Selenium: Supplementation of the diet with selenium might reduce the risk for developing breast cancer. Women with low blood levels of selenium have twice the cancer risk of women who have high blood levels of selenium. Low vitamin A status increases this risk. Selenium levels might be an indicator of future risk for cancer.[58,66]

Selenium might offer some protection against breast cancer, however, it cannot counteract the harmful effects of a high-fat diet. A reduction in dietary fat and an adequate intake of selenium are necessary in the prevention of breast cancer.[67]

Selenium is found in lean meats, whole grain breads and cereals, seafood, and mushrooms. The selenium content of the food depends on the selenium content of the soil in which the food is grown. If

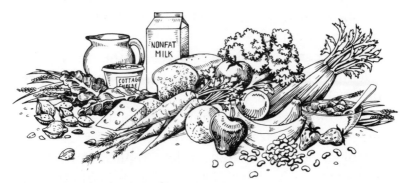

Figure 6. The Vegetarian Diet

plants are grown and cattle are raised on selenium-rich soil, then the foods will be good sources. Foods grown in selenium-poor regions will contribute little selenium to the diet. Lean meats and seafood are a more reliable source of selenium because the mineral is concentrated in the tissues of animals and seafoods. A daily intake of 50 to 200 mcg is considerd safe and adequate for most healthy people. Since meats and seafoods are especially rich in selenium and there is a great variability of selenium in plant foods, vegetarians and people who consume limited amounts of meat would probably benefit from a supplement of 50 to 100 mcg/day.[68] If the supplement contains the inorganic form of selenium, sodium selenite, it should not be taken with vitamin C. Vitamin C taken at the same time as sodium selenite might impair the absorption of selenium.[99]

Breast Self-Exam: Every woman more than 20 years old should perform a monthly breast self-exam. If the exam becomes a normal part of a woman's health care, she will become familiar with the normal shape and irregularities of the breast and can more accurately detect an abnormal or new growth.

The breasts should be examined the first week following the menstrual period. Important changes to note are lumps that do not expand and shrink with different stages of the menstrual cycle, are not tender to touch, and are harder than other lumps.

A woman should consult a physician if any lump or change in the breast tissue is noted. When cancer is detected and treated in the early stages the chances of survival and a return to health are greatly improved. The survival rate is 100% if the cancer is detected before the tumor has invaded surrounding tissue.[69]

Other Cancers

Endometrial And Ovarian Cancer: Obesity is the single most important risk factor in the development of endometrial and ovarian cancer. About 65% of all women with this disease have a history of obesity, high blood cholesterol levels, and elevated levels of estrogen.[65,70]

Dietary fat also increases the risk of endometrial cancer. In a study comparing the incidence of this form of cancer in 23 countries, the United States population had the highest rate of cancer of the endometrium, as well as the highest fat consumption. Fatty foods associated with this increased risk are meats, shortening and butter, and vegetable oils.[65]

Cervical Cancer: Unlike cancers of the breast, endometrium, and ovary that are related to excesses in dietary fat and body weight, cervical cancer appears to be related to dietary deficiencies. Dietary intake of vitamin A and beta carotene, the plant form of vitamin A, is low in women who develop cervical cancer as compared to healthy women. Vitamin A is essential for the normal growth of epithelial tissue, the type of tissue that covers all internal and external surfaces of the body, including the cervix. This fat-soluble vitamin also might be important in the maintenance of a healthy immune system.[71]

Dietary intake of at least the RDA for vitamin A, 4,000 IU, is recommended for all healthy women. This recommendation is based on the prevention of classic vitamin A deficiency and might not be adequate to prevent the development of cancer. Larger daily doses of 10,000 IU to 25,000 IU have been suggested to decrease the risk of cancer.[72] *(Figure 7, Page 33)*

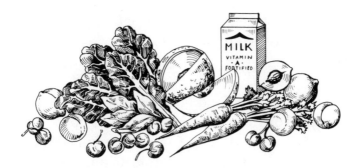

Figure 7.   Foods High In Vitamin A

Vitamin A as retinol in supplementation form might produce side effects at doses exceeding 25,000 IU to 50,000 IU. In larger doses, vitamin A can be toxic. The beta carotene form of vitamin A is not toxic to adults; except for a temporary yellowing of the skin that recedes when the dose is lessened, large amounts can be consumed with no apparent harm.[73]

Vitamin C also might help prevent cervical cancer. A low vitamin C intake is more common in women with cervical abnormalities and cancer. Women whose intake of vitamin C is less than 88 mg/day are 4.35 times more likely to develop cervical abnormalities or cancer. Women who consume 30 mg a day (one-half the RDA) might have a sevenfold increase in risk of cervical abnormalities as compared to women who consume at least the RDA. Protection from cervical abnormalities is associated with higher intakes of vitamin C, especially intakes of 88 mg/day or more. National nutrition surveys show that vitamin C intake is low in the United States population and 20% to 40% of all women consume less than 70% of the Recommended Dietary Allowance.[71,74]

Although vitamin C intake is a risk factor for cervical cancer, it is not independent of vitamin A. The conversion of beta carotene to vitamin A (retinol) is dependent on vitamin C. Both nutrients are needed for protection from cervical abnormalities and cancer.[71] *(Figure 8)*

The B vitamin folic acid also is important in the normal growth of cervical tissue. Foods that are good sources of vitamin C also supply folic acid and the association between vitamin C and cervical cancer might be linked to the folic acid in the food.[75]

A low-fat, high-fiber diet reduces a woman's risk for developing cancer. This diet is low in fatty meat and dairy products; prepared or convenience foods that contain oils, gravies, sauces, or other fats; and vegetable oils. The diet is high in fruits and vegetables, whole grain breads and cereals, dried beans and peas, nonfat or low-fat dairy foods, poultry, and fish. Vitamins A, C, and folic acid are supplied by fruits and dark green leafy vegetables. Several servings should be included in the diet each day.[76]

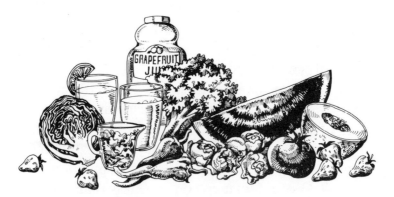

Figure 8. Foods High In Vitamin C

5
Osteoporosis

What Is Osteoporosis?

Osteoporosis is a degenerative bone disease characterized by the loss of calcium from the bones over a prolonged period of time. As a result, bones become brittle and are easily fractured.

Back pain and a loss of height resulting from compressed, weakened vertebrae are classic symptoms of advanced osteoporosis. The spinal deformity commonly known as Dowager's Hump results when vertebra are compressed. In addition, weakened bones are prone to spinal fractures that can occur with otherwise harmless events such as coughing, stepping from a curb, or receiving an overly aggressive hug.[77] *(Figure 9, Page 36)*

Osteoporosis is usually the underlying cause for the 190,000 broken hips among senior citizens each year. In addition, a majority of the one million bone fractures that occur annually are attributed to osteoporosis.[78]

Osteoporosis is most common in older women, although men also can suffer from the disease. The hormonal changes that accompany menopause hasten calcium loss from the bones. Calcium loss is most pronounced during the first few years after menopause. Although bone loss usually continues, it does so at a slower rate.[79]

Women who are most vulnerable are those who enter menopause with less than optimal bone density. It is easier to prevent osteoporosis than to treat it. Positive dietary and lifestyle habits started at an early

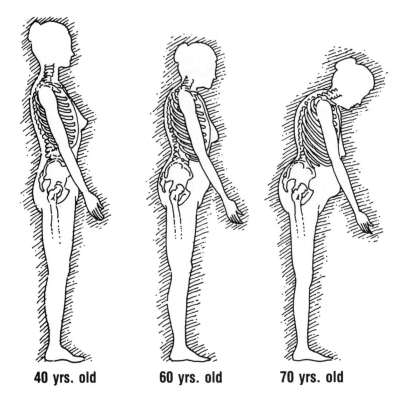

| 40 yrs. old | 60 yrs. old | 70 yrs. old |

Figure 9.   The Development Of Osteoporosis

When vertebrae are weakened by osteoporosis, they collapse and cause a loss of height, curvature of the spine, and a protruding abdomen.

age and continued throughout life will help protect bones from the devastating effects of the disease.

Bones are active tissues. Calcium is added to and removed from bone every day. The process is called bone remodeling. When calcium deposition is greater than calcium loss, bones grow stronger. If the two processes occur at an even rate, bone is maintained. When calcium loss exceeds calcium deposition, bones become increasingly brittle. Continued calcium loss often leads to osteoporosis.

Diet And Bone Density

While a woman attains her adult height early in life, her bones continue to grow in density until she is in her 30s, provided she consumed a high calcium diet to that point. Women entering middle age with strong bones are less likely to suffer from osteoporosis later in life.[80,81]

Although the Recommended Dietary Allowance (RDA) for calcium is 800 mg daily, recent studies indicate that premenopausal women need approximately 1,000 mg daily and postmenopausal women between 1,200 mg and 1,700 mg daily.[79] Three servings of milk or cheese plus a variety of other foods provides the recommended calcium intake for the premenopausal woman.

Many women avoid dairy products because milk and cheese are considered high-fat foods. However, nonfat and low-fat diary products supply as much calcium as their high-fat counterparts.

Concern about weight control has made many women avoid milk, yet three glasses of nonfat milk provide only 250 calories. Low-fat and whole milk would provide 420 and 450 calories, respectively. Women intolerant to lactose, the natural sugar found in milk, can often tolerate yogurt and cheese since these foods are lower in lactose.

Calcium Supplements

A variety of calcium supplements are available. Calcium carbonate is the least expensive and supplies the highest amount of calcium per tablet. The concentration of calcium in calcium gluconate is small. Many tablets would have to be taken during the day to obtain an adequate dose. The absorption of calcium from calcium lactate is better than from calcium carbonate. However, the percentage of calcium in the lactate form is almost as low as that from the gluconate form. Women with lactose intolerance should avoid calcium lactate.[82] *(Table 6)*

Although bone meal and dolomite are high in calcium, they may contain lead and other toxic metals and should be avoided, unless the products can be proven to be free of contamination.[83.]

Vitamin D

Vitamin D is essential for the absorption of calcium and an adequate dietary intake is important for the maintenance of healthy bones. Even though vitamin D can be produced in the body when a person is exposed to sunlight, women who live in cloudy or smoggy environments as well as women who stay indoors most of the time would benefit from a sup-

Table 6.	Calcium Content Of Supplements		
Supplement	Percent Calcium	Example Dose (mg)	Amount of Calcium (mg)
Calcium carbonate	40%	1,200 mg	480 mg
Calcium phosphate	32%	1,200 mg	384 mg
Calcium lactate	18%	1,200 mg	216 mg
Calcium gluconate	9%	1,200 mg	108 mg

plement. The body is less efficient at manufacturing vitamin D as a person ages and dietary sources of the vitamin become more important in the later years.[84]

The Recommended Dietary Allowance for vitamin D is 400 IU/day, the amount of vitamin D in one quart of vitamin D-fortified milk. Other dairy foods, such as yogurt, cheese, sour cream, or cottage cheese do not contain appreciable amounts of vitamin D.

The American Society for Bone and Mineral research recommends avoiding amounts of vitamin D in excess of 1,000 IU per day.[85] Vitamin D in large doses might cause nausea, weakness, headache, digestive disturbances, irreversible kidney and heart damage, and calcification of soft tissue, which is the deposition of calcium into tissues such as the kidney.

Estrogen And Osteoporosis

Estrogen replacement therapy helps prevent bone loss in women who have had "surgical menopause," the surgical removal of the ovaries or have gone through natural menopause. Estrogen replacement helps prevent premature bone loss. A recommended estrogen dosage for menopausal women is between 0.3 and 0.625 mg/day for 21 days and supplemented on days 17 through 21 with a progestational agent. While estrogen therapy is helpful in reducing bone loss, the combination of calcium and estrogen appears to be more effective.[79]

Estrogen should only be taken with the supervision of a physician. The concern in estrogen therapy is the effect of estrogen on the increased risk for developing some forms of cancer. The combination of a low-dose estrogen and a progestational agent, however, might reduce the risk for developing cancer.[79]

Other Lifestyle Factors

Protein: Americans consume too much protein. Actual protein requirements are low compared to typical protein intake. The Recommended Dietary Allowance (RDA) for women is 44 grams per day. A turkey sandwich (3 1/2 ounces of turkey, 2 slices of whole wheat bread), a glass of nonfat milk, and potato salad provide more than a woman's daily requirement for protein. A high protein diet causes an increased urinary excretion of calcium. The dietary intake of calcium must be increased to compensate for the loss.[86]

Alcohol: Excessive alcohol consumption has a negative effect on calcium balance. Alcohol interferes with the absorption of calcium, even when supplements of vitamin D are provided.[86]

Coffee: Coffee also might contribute to a calcium deficiency. Postmenopausal women with osteoporosis tend to consume more coffee than women of the same age with healthy bones. Whether coffee consumption causes the bone loss or is a contributor to the disorder has not been substantiated, however a possible link between coffee and bone loss is suggested.[87]

Cigarettes: Smoking promotes the loss of calcium from the bone.[85]

Fiber: Excess consumption of dietary fiber or unleavened whole wheat products might interfere with calcium absorption. This is especially true of cereal fibers such as bran that are high in phytates. Phytates are compounds in whole wheat that bind to some minerals in the intestine and reduce their absorption. Phytates are not a problem in leavened whole wheat products, such as bread, since these whole grain products contain an enzyme called phytase that deactivates phytates.[85]

Physical Activity: Pressure on the bones and resistance to the force of gravity is essential for the maintenance of bone strength. Weight bearing activity, such as walking, running, aerobic dancing, jumping rope, and tennis, is essential for maintaining the balance between calcium loss and calcium deposition in the bone. Exercise can stimulate the growth of new bone, even in elderly women who follow a program of mild exercise and physical therapy. Aerobic dancing and walking increases bone width in younger postmenopausal women and weight bearing activity may be effective in preventing postmenopausal osteoporosis.[77,85,88]

While exercise is beneficial, excessive exercise might have a negative effect on bone mass. Preliminary research indicates that premenopausal women who work out excessively and who subsequently cease menstruating have a bone mass 22% to 30% below menstruating women.[89]

Stress: Stress interferes with calcium absorption, increases calcium excretion, and might contribute to the development of osteoporosis.[90]

In summary, a diet throughout life that contains ample amounts of calcium and vitamin D, that provides adequate but not excessive fiber and protein, and includes reduced consumption of coffee and alcohol is the best defense against osteoporosis. In addition, moderate physical activity and not smoking will further reduce a woman's risk for this bone disorder. (See CALCIUM AND NUTRITION, published by Health Media of America, Inc.)

6
Weight Control

Many women, in an effort to lose weight, drastically reduce calories or follow one of the many popular current diets. Many of these current diets are nutritionally unsound and provide less than the recommended amounts of vitamins, minerals, fiber, or other nutrients. Quick weight loss is seldom maintained. The dieter loses ten pounds in one week, resumes previous eating habits, and gains the weight that was lost. More than a two to four pound weight loss per week indicates that more fluid and protein from muscle and other lean tissues is lost than fat.

When total caloric intake falls below 1,500 calories, adequate nutrition is difficult and supplementation might be necessary.[91]

A woman should carefully assess her weight history and current weight before a diet is planned. A realistic weight goal that can be attained and maintained must be determined. If a woman has been heavy throughout life, it might be unrealistic to try to reach and maintain a thin body size.

For the woman who needs to lose weight and maintain that weight loss, a reduced calorie diet of not less than 1,200 calories is recommended. Two of every three food selections should be fresh fruits and vegetables, whole grain breads and cereals, and dried beans and peas. A minimum of two servings of non-fat milk or yogurt and lean meat, chicken, or fish is necessary. Foods should be baked, steamed, or broiled. Sauces, gravies, and other fatty foods should be avoided. *(Table 7, Page 45)*

The diet must be individualized, realistic, and practical. The diet will only be effective if it is accompanied by a personalized, routine aerobic exercise program, such as walking, jogging, aerobic dance, jumping rope, swimming, or bicycling. For women over 35 years old, a physical examination by a physician is recommended before initiating a weight control/exercise program.

A modified, supplemented fast has been effective for some women who have more than 50 pounds to lose. This type of weight loss program should be used with the guidance of a physician. An important component of a weight loss program is a well-structured, follow-up program that stresses the need for continued support and provides guidelines for weight maintenance.[92]

Vitamin-mineral supplementation might be necessary for a woman who consumes less than 1,500 calories a day. Guidelines for choosing a supplement include:

- Choose a multiple vitamin-mineral that contains vitamin A, vitamin D, vitamin E, vitamin B_1, vitamin B_2, niacin, vitamin B_6, vitamin B_{12}, folic acid, pantothenic acid, biotin, chromium, copper, iron, magnesium, manganese, molybdenum, selenium, and zinc.
- Choose a supplement that provides between one and three times the USRDA for each vitamin or mineral. Few multiple vitamin-mineral prepara-

Table 7   Cutting Back On Fat And Calories

Instead of . . .	Use . . .
☑ Whole milk	☐ Nonfat or low-fat milk
☑ Doughnuts, pastry, cake, pie	☐ Bagel, English muffin (whole wheat)
☑ Cheese (Cheddar, American, Swiss, etc.)	☐ Low fat cheeses
	☐ Nuts
☑ Bacon, sausage	☑ Turkey
☑ Potato chips, corn chips	☑ Whole grain crackers, Unbuttered popcorn
☐ Hard margarine	☑ Soft margarine or butter
☐ Sour cream	☐ Low fat yogurt
☑ Soda, fruit drinks	☑ Fruit juice, water
☐ White bread, & white bread products	☑ Whole grain bread & whole grain products
☑ Luncheon meats, hot dogs	☐ Fresh, frozen or canned fish
☐ Heavily marbled or fatty beef, pork	☐ Lean beaf, veal, chicken, turkey
☐ Hamburger, with more than 20% fat	☐ Lean hamburger
☑ Sugar-coated cereals	☐ Whole grain, ''plain'' cereals
☑ Candy, cookies	☐ Raisins, dried fruit
☑ Tuna packed in oil	☐ Water-packed tuna
☑ Fruit, canned or frozen in syrup	☐ Fresh or frozen unsweetened fruit

Count the checks in each column. If you have more checks in the left hand column than in the right, your total diet is probably too high in fat, salt, or sugar to be healthy for you.

tions contain the USRDA for calcium and magnesium and a separate supplement of these nutrients might be required to meet daily needs.

Eating Disorders

Fear of obesity causes some women to skip meals, eat unbalanced diets, or consume limited food at each meal. In girls, these eating patterns can retard growth and delay puberty.[93]

This fear of obesity is different from anorexia, a serious eating disorder characterized by a distorted body image, self-imposed starvation, excessive preoccupation with not eating, and compulsive exercise.[94]

Women of all ages can suffer from this obsession with eating and starvation. Women with anorexia jeopardize their nutritional status and overall health.

The eating patterns of bulimic women fluctuate between excessive food intake and restricted food intake. Bulimic women can eat an average of 4,500 calories daily and vomit repetitively and/or abuse laxatives to rid themselves of huge quantities of food. When bulimics eat a limited amount of food their diets are inadequate in fiber, potassium, calcium, magnesium, iron, and vitamin B_1. Additional loss of nutrients results from induced vomiting and diarrhea.[94]

Symptoms of abnormal eating behaviors include preoccupation with food, eating, fear of weight gain, or avoidance of eating; an attempt to maintain weight below suggested values; daily weighing with rigid food restriction when body weight increases as little as one-half pound; self-induced vomiting after meals; fluctuations between binging and fasting or semi-starvation; a belief that more weight needs to be lost in spite of comments by others that the person is too thin; amenorrhea (cessation of the menstrual cycle); excessive exercise; and extraordinary pride in self-denial. One of these symptoms does not indicate anorexia or bulimia, but a combination of several behaviors suggests that a woman's attitude toward eating and food might not be normal.

Education in meal selection, nutrition, and normal eating behaviors is only one part of the treatment for anorexia and bulimia. Altering compulsive eating behaviors might require counseling from a professional and support from family and friends.

7
Other Health Concerns Of Women

Nutrition For The Physically Active Woman

The nutritional needs of the recreational exerciser (non-competition athlete) are similar to the general guidelines for healthy eating except food intake might be greater to meet the increased calorie demands of regular exercise. At least 55% of calories should come from complex carbohydrates, 30% of calories from fats, and 12% from protein. Whole grain breads and cereals will supply added amounts of B vitamins, trace minerals, and fiber that are not found in white or enriched grains.

An important difference in dietary recommendations is the fluid requirement. The woman who exercises regularly, whether it is jogging, lifting weights, aerobic dance, swimming, tennis, golf, or any other sport, loses water in perspiration. The thirst sensation is a poor indicator of water loss and a woman may quench her thirst and still be dehydrated. Chronic inadequate intake of water can affect general health, the softness of skin, and can place a woman at increased risk for heat exhaustion.

A general guideline for replacing fluid losses is to drink twice as much water as quenches the thirst, or drink one pint of water for every pound lost during exercise. This requires weighing before and after each exercise session. The best fluid replacement is water, but fruit or vegetable juices are nutritious alternatives. Salt tablets are not recommeded. Even if a woman does not exercise, 6 to 8 glasses of water should be consumed each day.

Some evidence suggests that vigorous exercise and training might increase a woman's need for some vitamins and minerals. Increased urinary loss of the trace minerals chromium and zinc are found in some athletes with a subsequent decline in blood levels of these minerals. The RDA for vitamin B_2 might not be adequate to maintain normal levels in women athletes.[95,96]

Anemia can result from vigorous training and is thought to be caused by the excessive pounding and jarring of the body in sports such as running combined with normal menstrual losses and poor dietary intake of iron. The inclusion of iron-rich foods is important for all women, especially those engaged in physical activity.[97]

Nutrition And Menopause

The nutritional needs of women during menopause are poorly understood and the nutritional recommendations are similar to the general guidelines for healthy eating. Although a woman's risk for cardiovascular disease has been less than a man's up to this point, after menopause the risk increases and by age 65 a woman's risk for atherosclerosis, heart attack, and stroke exceeds a man's risk. The general dietary guidelines are to consume two-thirds of the diet as foods from plant sources such as whole grain breads and cereals, dried beans and peas, vegetables, and fruits; maintain fat intake at no more than 30% of calories; consume a high fiber diet; limit intake of sugar and alcohol; and maintain desirable weight.[98]

The rate of bone loss escalates during and after menopause. Adequate calcium intake is necessary throughout life to prevent osteoporosis and daily intake of calcium might need to be increased to 1,200 mg to 1,700 mg after menopause. (See Section 5 on Osteoporosis.)

Summary

Nutrition is important in a woman's health. It does more than give her "get up and go." The foods a woman chooses might protect the tissues such as the breast, cervix, and endometrium from cancer. A nutritious diet can help decrease the depression often associated with use of birth control pills, assist in improving or eliminating the distressing symptoms of premenstrual syndrome, and prevent the crippling effects of osteoporosis.

Throughout life, attention to special nutritional needs is a woman's best defense against disease.

Appendix: Good Nutrition For The Woman On The Go

Women today are busier than they have ever been. It is often too easy to skip meals or choose convenience rather than nutrition. However, if a woman has time to grab a snack from a vending machine or grab a hamburger at a drive-through fast-food restaurant she has time to eat well. Good food can be prepared in minutes while still being enjoyable.

- Keep easy-to-prepare foods available. Fill the cupboards with low-fat crackers, beans, fruits canned in their own juice, tuna packed in water, and fruit juices. Keep fresh fruits and vegetables in the refrigerator, frozen vegetables and low-fat convenience entrees in the freezer, and whole grained

51

breads, such as pita bread, bagels, and bran muffins in the bread box.

- Prepare large quantities of foods ahead of time and store them in individual containers in the freezer. For example, homemade soups, stews, casseroles, spaghetti sauce and other low-fat sauces, cooked beans, brown rice, and sandwich spreads can be made and frozen for use later. Basic sauces can be thawed and seasoned several ways during the week. A pot of beans can be used throughout the week in salads, soups, pocket bread sandwiches, or mashed for "refried" beans wrapped in a tortilla. Make an extra serving for dinner and use the leftovers for lunch the next day. Prepare and freeze sandwiches or snacks for later use.
- Prepare simple meals. Lunch and dinner do not need to be elaborate. Combine three of the following four food groups at each meal:
  - Low-fat dairy products,
  - Fresh fruits and vegetables,
  - Whole grain breads or cereals, and /or
  - Low fat meat, chicken, fish, or dried beans and peas.

Sample menus:

Breakfast: Broil 1 slice whole wheat bread with farmer's cheese, a dash of cinnamon, and nutmeg. Serve with fruit juice or half of a cantaloupe.

OR

Breakfast: 1 package of instant oatmeal with non-fat milk, a banana, and raisins.

Lunch: Pita pocket bread with beans, tomatoes, cheese, sprouts, and green onions. Salad (make a large bowl and use throughout week), tomato juice.

OR

Lunch: Turkey slices and lettuce on whole wheat bread, nonfat milk, apple, nuts.

Dinner: Homemade soup or vegetable stew, brown bread, sliced vegetables.

OR

Dinner: Fresh fruit slices, cottage cheese, whole wheat rolls, slice of lean beef, rice or noodles.

- Snacks can be nutritious mini-meals:
  - A half of a papaya filled with nonfat yogurt.
  - Two rice cakes with peanut butter.
  - Strawberries, oranges, bananas, grapes.
  - Slice of whole wheat bread with apple slices and ricotta cheese.
  - Ready-to-eat cereal, such as spoon-sized Shredded Wheat.
  - Milkshake made with nonfat milk and fruit.
  - Air-popped popcorn.
  - Raw vegetables, such as carrots, jicama, celery, broccoli, zuccini, mushrooms, tomatoes, radishes, cabbage.
- Bag lunches can be easy and nutritious:
  - Use lean meats, chicken, low-fat cheeses, water-packed tuna or salmon, or beans for sandwich fillers. (Avoid cold cuts, sausage, liverwurst, and bologna).
  - Take a thermos of homemade soup or stew, spaghetti, a casserole, or leftovers.

- Try fruit and vegetables and nonfat yogurt dips.
- Take pasta salad with low-calorie dressing.
- Beverages can include nonfat milk, fruit juices, vegetable juices, carbonated or mineral water, or water.
- Use whole grain breads, bagels, rolls, muffins, tortillas (filled with beans, low-fat cheese, or cottage cheese and vegetables).

- Use kitchen equipment that will save time such as microwaves, crock pots, blenders, electric mixers, dishwashers, or food processors.
- Use commercial convenience foods with caution. Check the labels and avoid foods that contain more than 3 grams of fat for every 100 calories. Words such as "lite" do not guarantee the food is low in fat or calories.
- Plan ahead. Do not leave the house without a snack or meal for the day. Carry low-calorie, low-fat foods in a purse, briefcase, or glove compartment. Keep crackers and peanut butter or fresh fruit in a drawer of the desk at work. Keep nutritious snacks at home.

Dining Out

When ordering in restaurants:

- Choose salad bars or order salads with dressing on the side. Liquid dressings such as oil and vinegar coat the vegetables more evenly and less dressing can be used as compared to creamy dressings such as Thousand Island or Blue Cheese dressings.

- Ask how foods are prepared. Ask for meats and vegetables to be baked, steamed, or broiled without butter.
- Remove the skin from chicken.
- Avoid the following terms on the menu: refried, creamed, cream sauce, au gratin, cheese sauce, escalloped, au lait, a la mode, prime, au fromage, hollandaise, crispy, and sauteed.
- Choose whole grain breads and pastas when available.
- Choose desserts such as gelatin, fruit ices, fresh fruits, or angel food cake.
- Order ala carte or split an entree.
- Have extra food wrapped to take home.
- Ask for the plate to be removed to avoid the temptation of overeating.
- When on the road, ask for room service and tailor-make the meal to individual taste; request a special meal ahead of time from the airline; ask a native or the hotel concierge to recommend a restaurant that serves nutritious, low-fat meals; bring exercise clothes and take advantage of pools, spas, running paths, and local sites; and walk to appointments or activities.

References

1. Loeb M: America in the 1980's: 10 major changes ahead. *J Am Diet Assoc* 1981; 78:228-234.
2. Pao M, Mickle S: Problem nutrients in the United States. *Food Technology* 1981; 35:58-69.
3. Anderson R, Kozlovsky A: Chromium intake, absorption and excretion of subjects consuming self-selected diets. *Am J Clin Nutr* 1985; 41:1177-1183.
4. Tamura T: Folic acid. *Nutr & MD* 1984; 10:1-3.
5. *Ideas for Better Eating.* Menus and recipes to make use of the Dietary Guidelines, Science and Education Administration/Human Nutrition, US Dept of Agriculture, Jan 1981.
6. *Healthy People: The Surgeon General's Report on Health Promotion and Disease Prevention, 1979.* US Department of Health, Education, and Welfare, Washington DC, US Governement Printing Office, Publ. No 79-55071.
7. National Research Council: *Diet, Nutrition, and Cancer, 1982.* National Academy Press, 2101 Constitution Avenue, NW Washington DC, 20418.
8. Krause M, Mahan K: *Food, Nutrition and Diet Therapy* 7 ed. Philadelphia, WB Saunders Co, 1984, pp 585-599.
9. *Recommended Dietary Allowances,* 9 ed. Committee on Dietary Allowances, Food and Nutrition Board, National Research Council. Washington DC, National Academy of Sciences, 1980, pp 137-143.
10. Goodhart R, Shils M (eds): *Modern Nutrition in Health and Disease.* Philadelphia, Lea and Febiger, 1980, pp 324-354.
11. Garrison R, Somer E: *The Nutrition Desk Reference.* New Canaan, Conn, Keats Publishing Co, 1985, pp 66-67.
12. Feinstein R, Daniel W: Anemia and anemia in adolescents: value in screening examinations for sports. *Phys and Sportsmed* 1984; 12:140-144.
13. Loescher C: Female fitness, sports. *Nutr News* 1983; 1:1-3.
14. Bogert L, Briggs G, Calloway D: *Nutrition in Physical Fitness.* Philadelphia, W.B. Saunders, 1973, pp 263-272.

15. Hamilton E, Whitney E: *Nutrition: Concepts and Controversies* 2 ed. St Paul, West Publishing Co, 1982, p 326.
16. Hallberg L. Bioavailability of iron in man. *Ann Rev Nutr* 1981; 1:123-147.
17. Reed P: *Nutrition: An Applied Science.* St Paul, West Publishing Co, 1980, p 353.
18. Anderson P, Cumming C: *Nutritional Aberration, in Clinical Pharmacy and Therapeutics,* Herfindal E, Hirschman J (eds). Baltimore, Williams and Wilkins, 1979, pp 443.
19. Abraham G: Premenstrual tension. *Curr Prob in Obstet Gynecol* 1980; 3:5-8.
20. Dalton, K. *The Premenstrual Syndrome and Progesterone Therapy.* Chicago, Year Book Medical Publishers, 1984, pp 10-38.
21. Fuchs N, Hakim M, Abraham G: The effect of a nutritional supplement, Optivite for Women, on premenstrual tension syndromes. I: Effect on blood chemistry and serum steriod levels during the midluteal phase. *J Appl Nutr* 1985; 37:1-11.
22. Chakmakjian Z, Higgins C, Abraham G: The effect of a nutritional supplement, Optivite for Women, on premenstrual tension syndromes. II. Effect on symptomatology, using a double blind cross-over design.*J Appl Nutr* 1985; 37:12-17.
23. Goldin B, Aldercruetz H, Gorbach S, et al: Estrogen excretion patterns and plasma levels in vegetarian and omniverous women. *N Eng J Med* 1982; 307:1542-1547
24. Abraham G: Nutrition and the premenstrual tension syndromes. *J Appl Nutr* 1984; 36:103-124.
25. Abraham G:Nutritional factors in the etiology of the premenstrual tension syndromes. *J Repro Med* 1983; 28:446-464.
26. Seelig M: Magnesium requirements in human nutrition. *Cont Nutr* 1982; 7:1-2.
27. Abraham G, Lubran M: Serum and red cell magnesium levels in patients with premenstrual syndrome. *A J Clin Nutr* 1981; 34:2364-2366.

28. Goei G, Ralston J, Abraham G: Dietary patterns of patients with premenstrual syndrome. *J Appl Nutr* 1982; 34:4.
29. Barr W: Pyridoxine supplements in premenstrual syndrome. *Practitioner* 1984; 228:425-427.
30. Abraham G, Hargrove J: Effect of vitamin B_6 on premenstrual symptomatology in women with premenstrual tension syndromes: A double blind crossover study. *Infertility* 1980; 3:155-165.
31. Abraham G, Schwartz U, Lubran M: Effect of vitamin B_6 on plasma and red cell magnesium levels in premenopausal women. *Ann Clin Lab Sci* 1981; 11:333-336.
32. Schaumberg H, Kaplan J, Windebank A, et al: Sensory neuropathy from pyridoxine abuse. *N Eng J Med* 1983; 309:445.
33. Vitamin B_6 toxicity: A new megavitamin syndrome. *Nutr Rev* 1984; 42:44-46.
34. Brush M, Watson S, Horrobin D, et al: Abnormal essential fatty acid levels in plasma of women with premenstrual syndrome. *Am J Obstet Gynecol* 1984; 150:363-366.
35. Horrobin D: The role of essential fatty acids and prostaglandins in the premenstrual syndrome. *J Repro Med* 1983; 28:465-468.
36. Lindemann J: Premenstrual syndrome — A practical approach. *Wisconsin Med J* 1984; 83:30-32.
37. Loebl S, Spratto G, Wit A: *The Nurse's Handbook.* New York, John Wiley and Sons, 1977, pp 593-595.
38. Worthington-Roberts B, Vermeersch J, Williams S: *Nutrition in Pregnancy and Lactation.* St.Louis, Times Mirror/Mosby College Publishing, 1985, pp 371-395.
39. Adams P, Rose D, Folkard V, et al: Effect of pyridoxine hydrochloride (Vitamin B_6) upon depression associated with oral contraception. *Lancet* 1973; I:897.
40. Bosse T, Donald E: The vitamin B_6 requirement in oral contraceptive users.I. Assessment by pyridoxal level and transferase activity in erythrocytes. *Am J Clin Nutr* 1979; 32:1015-1023.

41. Lindenbaum J, Whitehead N, Reyner F: Oral contraceptive hormones, folate metabolism and the cervical epithelium. *Am J Clin Nutr* 1975; 28:346-353.
42. Butterworth C: New concepts in nutrition and cancer: Implications for folic acid. *Cont Nutr* 1980; 5.
43. Check W: Folate for oral contraceptive users may reduce cervical cancer risk. *JAMA* 1980; 244:633-634.
44. Tamura T, Shane B, Baer M, et al: Absorption of mono- and polyglutamate folates in zinc-depleted man. *A J Clin Nutr* 1978; 31:1984-1987.
45. Thorp V: Effect of oral contraceptive agents on vitamin and mineral requirements. *J Am Diet Assoc* 1980; 76:581-584.
46. Hutter R: Goodbye to fibrocystic disease. *N Eng J Med* 1985; 312:179-181.
47. Love S, Gelman R, Silen W: Fibrocystic "disease" of the breast - a non-disease? *N Eng J Med* 1982; 307:1010-1014.
48. Hutter R: Goodbye to fibrocystic disease. *N Eng J Med* 1985; 312:179-181.
49. Minton J, Foecking M, Webster D, et al: Caffeine, cyclic nucleotides and breast disease. *Surgery* 1979; 86:105-109.
50. Wenneker M: Breast lumps: is caffeine the culprit? *Nutr Action* 1980; 7:3-6.
51. Brooks P, Gart S, Heldfond A, et al: Measuring the effect of caffeine restriction on fibrocystic breast disease. *J Repro Med* 1981; 26:279-282.
52. Snowdon D, Phillips R: Coffee consumption and risk of fatal cancers. *Am J Public Health* 1984; 74:820-823.
53. Haffner S, Knapp J, Stern M, et al: Coffee consumption, diet, and lipids. *Am J Epidem* 1985; 122:1-12.
54. Vitamin E for cystic breast disease: Effect on homeostasis. *JAMA* 1980; 244:1077-1080.
55. Jick H: Coffee and myocardial infarction. *New Eng J Med* 1973; 289:63.
56. Rose D, Boyer A, Haley N, et al: Low fat diet in fibrocystic disease of the breast with cyclical mastalgia: A feasibility study. *Am J Clin Nutr* 1985; 41:856.

57. Newell G, Ellison N (eds): *Nutrition and Cancer: Etiology and Treatment.* New York, Raven Press, 1981, pp 93-110.

58. Committee on Diet, Nutrition and Cancer, Assembly of Life Sciences, National Research Council: *Diet, Nutrition and Cancer.* Washington, DC, National Academy Press, 1982.

59. Kelsey J: A review of the epidemiology of human breast cancer. *Epidemiolog Rev* 1979; 1:74-109.

60. Erickson K, Deem R, Young L: Relationship of dietary fat to mammary hyperplastic alveolar nodule tumorigenesis and immune response. *Fed Proc* 1985; 44:1672.

61. Chow C: Nutritional influence on cellular antioxidant defense systems. *Am J Clin Nutr* 1979; 32:1066-1081.

62. Baumgartner W: Antioxidants, cancer and the immune response, in Kharasch N: *Trace Metals in Health and Disease.* New York, Raven Press, 1979, pp 297-302.

63. Horwitt M: *Vitamin E, in Modern Nutrition in Health and Disease* 6 ed, Goodhard R, Shils M (eds), Lea and Febiger, Philadelphia, 1980, pp 187.

64. *Dietary Goals for the United States* 2 ed. Select Committee on Nutrition and Human Needs, United States Senate, 1977. Washington DC, US Government Printing Office, Stock No 052-070-04376-8.

65. Simpoulos A: Fat intake, obesity and cancer of the breast and endometrium. *Med Oncol* 1985; 2:125-135.

66. Willett W, MacMahon B: Diet and cancer — An overview. *N Eng J Med* 1984; 310:697-703.

67. Ip C: Anticarcinogenic effect of selenium in the dimethylbenz(a)-anthracene-induced mammary tumor model in rats. *J Am Oil Chemists Soc* 1984; 61:1881.

68. Levander O: Selenium and chromium in human nutrition. *J Am Diet Assoc* 1975; 66:338-344.

69. *Cancer Facts and Figures 1985.* American Cancer Society, Inc, 90 Park Avenue, New York, NY 10016.

70. LaVecchia C, Franceschi S, Gallus G, et al: Oestrogens and obesity as risk factors for endometrial cancer in Italy. *Int J Epidemol* 1982; 11:120-126.

71. Romeny S, Palan P, Duttagupta C, et al: Retinoids and the prevention of cervical dysplasias. *Am J Obstet Gynecol* 1981; 141:890-894.
72. Kummet T, Meyskens F: Vitamin A: A potential inhibitor of human cancer. *Seminars in Oncology* 1983; 10:281.
73. *Recommended Dietary Allowances* 9 ed, Committee on Dietary Allowances, Food and Nutrition Board, National Research Council. Washington DC, National Academy of Sciences, 1980, pp 55-59.
74. Wassertheil-Smoller S: Low vitamin C intake as a risk for cervical dysplasia in Butterworth C, Hutchinson M (eds): *Nutritional Factors in the Induction and Maintenance of Malignancy,* Orlando, Academic Press, 1983, pp 289-301.
75. Bright-See E: Role of vitamins C and E in the etiology of human cancer in Prasad, K (ed) *Vitamins, Nutrition and Cancer,* Basel, Karger, 1984, pp 68-75.
76. Butterworth C, Norris D: Folic acid and vitamin C in cervical dysplasia. *Am J Clin Nutr* 1983; 37:332-333.
77. Marcus R: Calcium, skeletal aging and osteoporosis. *Nutr & M.D.* 1985; 11:1-3.
78. Jackson T, Ullrich I: Understanding osteoporosis. *Postgraduate Medicine* 1984; 75:119-125.
79. Ibid, pp 119-123.
80. Recker R: Osteoporosis. *Cont Nutr* 1983; 8:1-2.
81. Matkovic V, Kostial K, Simonovic I: Bone status and fracture rates in two regions of Yugoslavia. *Am J Clin Nutr* 1979; 32:540-549.
82. Calcium supplementation in adult women. *Nutr & M.D.* 1985; 11:1.
83. Advice on limiting intake of bonemeal. *Clin Pediatr* 1982; 21:590.
84. MacLaughlin J, Holick M: Aging decreases the capacity of human skin to produce vitamin D3. *J Clin Inv* 1985; 76:1536-1538.
85. Notelowvitz M, Ware M: *Stand Tall.* Gainesville, Triad Publishing, 1982, pp 88-113.
86. Allen L: Calcium bioavailability and absorption: A review. *Am J Clin Nutr* 1982; 35:783-808.
87. Notelowvitz M, Ware M: *Stand Tall.* Gainesville, Triad Publishing, 1982, p 102.

88. White M, Martin B, Yeater R, et al: The effects of exercise on the bones of postmenopausal women. *Int Orthoped* 1984; 7:209-214.
89. Lutter J: Mixed messages about osteoporosis in female athletes. *Physician and Sportsmed* 1983; 11:154-165.
90. Avioli L: Calcium and phosphorus, in Goodhart R, Shils M (eds): *Modern Nutrition in Health and Disease* 6 ed. Philadelphia, Lea and Febiger, 1980, p 300.
91. *Ideas for Better Eating,* USDA, January 1981.
92. Newton K: Weight management: Learning to self-regulate dietary habits. *Nutr Report* 1986; 4:12-16.
93. Unwarranted dieting retards growth and delays puberty. *Nutr Rev* 1984; 42:14-15.
94. Diets for treated bulimic patients. *Nutr & M.D.* 1985; 11:1.
95. Anderson R, Polansky M, Bryden N: Strenuous running: Acute effects of chromium, copper, zinc, and selected clinical variables in urine and serum of male runners. *Biol Trace El Res* 1984; 6:327-336.
96. Belko A, Obarzanek E, Roach R, et al: Effects of aerobic exercise and weight loss on riboflavin requirements of moderately obese, marginally deficient young women. *Am J Clin Nutr* 1984; 40:553-561.
97. Pate R: Sports anemia and its impact on athletic performance, in *Nutrition and Athletic Performance, Proceedings of the Conference on Nutritional Determinants in Athletic Performance,* San Francisco, September 24-25, 1981. Palo Alto, Bull Publishing Co, 1981, pp 202-217.
98. Roe D: *Drugs and Nutrition in the Geriatric Patient,* New York, Churchill Livingstone, 1984.
99. Robinson M, Huemmer P: Effect of a megadose of ascorbic acid, a meal and orange juice on the absorption of selenium as sodium selenite. *NZ Med J* 1985; 98:627-629.

Glossary

Aerobic Exercise: Physical activity that requires a constant supply of oxygen and uses large muscles groups in continuous motion. Examples of aerobic exercises are walking, bicycling, swimming, jogging, and jumping rope.

Anemia: A reduction in the number, size, or color of red blood cells; results in reduced oxygen- carrying capacity of the blood.

Anorexia: The lack or loss of appetite for food associated with weight loss and muscle wastage.

Antioxidant: A compound that protects other compounds or tissues from oxygen by reacting with oxygen.

Benign: Not harmful, not malignant.

Beta-carotene: The form of vitamin A found in plant foods such as carrots and dark green leafy vegetables.

Bulimia: An eating disorder characterized by excessive food intake followed by vomiting, laxative use, or fasting.

Cardiovascular: Pertaining to the heart and blood vessels.

Cervical: Pertaining to the cervix.

Cervix: The neck or necklike opening. Usually refers to the opening to the uterus.

Fetus: Unborn child still in the uterus.

Endometrium: The lining of the uterus.

Estrogen: A female hormone; steroid hormone produced and secreted by the ovaries.

Free Radical: A highly reactive compound derived from air pollution, radiation, cigarette smoke, or the incomplete breakdown of proteins and fats; reacts with fats in cell membranes and changes their shape or function.

Gastrointestinal: The stomach and intestinal tract.

Hematocrit: The volume percent of red blood cells in blood.

Heme Iron: Iron associated with hemoglobin in red blood cells. A form of iron found in meat, chicken, and fish that is well absorbed.

Hemoglobin: The oxygen-carrying protein in red blood cells.

Hormone: A chemical substance produced by an organ, called an endocrine gland, that is released into the blood and transported to another organ or tissue, where it performs a specific action. Examples of hormones are estrogen, adrenalin, and insulin.

Hyperhydration: Over accumulation of water in the body.

Hypertension: High blood pressure.

Immune System: A complex system of substances and tissues that protects the body from disease.

Lactation: Breastfeeding.

Lactose: The sugar found in milk.

Lesion: A damage to tissue caused by disease or injury.

Linoleic Acid: An essential polyunsaturated fatty acid that cannot be produced by the body and must be supplied from dietary sources such as vegetable oils.

Malignant: Cancerous.

Mastectomy: Surgical removal of a breast.

Menstruation: The monthly discharge of blood and tissue from the uterus.

Methylxanthines: Compounds in foods, such as theobromine in tea and chocolate, theophylline in tea, and caffeine in coffee. Methylxanthines might encourage fibrocystic breast disease in some women.

Non-Heme Iron: Iron found in foods from plant sources. Non-heme iron is more abundant than heme iron but is poorly absorbed.

Obesity: Body weight more than 20% above desirable weight; excessive fat.

Ovary: A glandular organ in the female reproductive system that produces the ovum (egg) and secretes the female hormones estrogen and progesterone.

Phytate: A compound in unleavened whole grains that binds to minerals in the intestine and inhibits their absorption.

Placebo: A medicine that has no pharmacological effect.

Polyunsaturated Fat: A type of unsaturated fat that is liquid at room temperature and is found in vegetable oils, nuts, seeds, and fish.

Postmenopausal: After the menopause.

Progesterone: A female hormone secreted by the ovaries.

Prolactin: A female hormone that stimulates the production of breastmilk.

66

Prostaglandin: A group of hormone-like substances formed from fatty acids that have profound effects on the body, including contraction and relaxation of smooth muscles and blood vessels.

Recommended Dietary Allowances (RDA): The amounts of nutrients recommended by the Food and Nutrition Board of the National Academy of Sciences to meet the needs of most healthy groups of people in the United States.

Serum: The fluid portion of blood that is left after the clotting factors have been removed. Serum is a straw colored fluid with red blood cells.

Vaginal: Pertaining to the vagina.

Index

70

Vitamin A, p 21, 30, 32-34, 44
   sources, p 20
Vitamin B_1, p 20, 44, 46
   sources, p 20
Vitamin B_2, p 20, 44, 50
   sources, p 20
Vitamin B_6, p 1, 2, 15, 17-20, 44, 50
Vitamin B_{12}, p 1, 2, 9, 10, 44
Vitamin C, p 1, 7, 8, 31, 33, 34
   sources, p 34
Vitamin D, p 38-41, 44
Vitamin E, p 2, 25-27, 44
   sources, p 27

W

Water, p 49, 50
Weight Control, p 3, 13, 37, 43-45
   and calories, p 43, 44, 45
   and exercise, p 44
   and fat, p 43
   and fiber, p 43
   and hyperhydration, p 13
   and menopause, p 50
   and protein, p 43

Z

Zinc, p 21, 44
   sources, p 21

Notes